Who Says Age Should Slow You Down?

John Molyneux

Moly Publishing

johnmolyneux.com

First published 2020 in the United Kingdom by Moly Publishing

ISBN 978-1-9161271-4-2 (print)
ISBN 978-1-9161271-5-9 (ebook)

A catalogue record for this book is available from the British Library

Printed in the United Kingdom

Cover design by Ken Leeder
Illustrations by Lydia Hughes
Interior design and layout by Daisy Editorial

Disclaimer

This book is not intended as a substitute for professional medical advice. The reader is advised to consult an appropriate healthcare professional regarding all aspects of individual healthcare. The author assumes no responsibility for loss or damage caused directly or indirectly by the use of information contained in this book. Individuals who suffer from any disease or are recovering from injury should consult with their doctor regarding the advisability of undertaking any of the exercises suggested in this book. The author disclaims any liability incurred from the use or application of the contents of this book.

Contents

About the author

John Molyneux has over 20 years' experience as a qualified and accredited sports therapist. He has developed a skill and passion for bringing exercise to those who struggle to maintain a regime or to exercise at all. He has particular expertise in working with age-related barriers, beginning with a gentle and appropriate introduction to exercise and gradually developing ability and confidence.

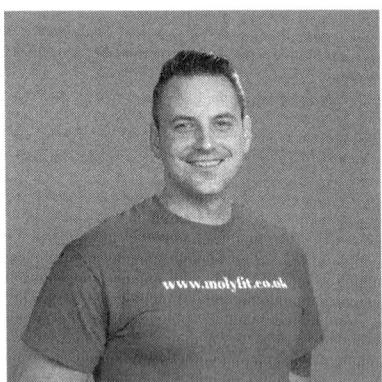

John firmly believes that exercise is accessible to anyone regardless of their age, ability or physical restrictions. This book is the product of his experience and is an easy-to-use guide for anyone who wants to acquire an exercise routine independently.

Safety

Most of these exercises are designed to be done on a bed, either sitting or standing. Occasionally, you will need to support your body weight. Ensure whatever you use is sturdy and stable and can support you. Wear comfortable clothes and appropriate, supportive footwear. Make sure the area you are working out in is free of trip hazards and obstructions.

Whilst exercising, if you experience chest pain, dizziness or severe shortness of breath then stop immediately and contact your doctor. If your symptoms do not go away when you stop exercising and you feel very unwell, contact your local health helpline without delay (in the UK dial 111) or call an ambulance.

If you experience pain in your muscles or joints, stop and check your technique then try again. If the pain persists, seek advice from a healthcare professional. It is normal to feel muscle soreness the next day and even 72 hours after exercise. That shows that the exercises are working.

Drink regular sips of water whilst you are exercising and when the exercise has finished.

Some of the exercises will work on your balance and coordination. If you have any doubt or hesitation before or during the exercise, make sure someone is there to help or support you during the exercise.

Don't forget to breathe! Take slow, deep breaths in and out whilst you are exercising.

Let's get you moving

Without a consultation and discussion about your full medical history, it would be irresponsible to promise that this book will definitely help you to walk unaided. However, I do think it is definitely worth a try!

Yes, we all slow with age. Yes, our muscles atrophy and naturally weaken each decade, but have you actually tried to fix the reason for needing a stick or walker? So many people I work with professionally who use sticks haven't. Sometimes a family member gave them a stick, or their doctor suggested it, or they just made the decision to use one without considering whether exercise could help. This book will challenge that decision. Over the next 20 weeks, we will look at all of the reasons why you might be walking with a stick, and with a few exercises each day, we will try to tackle those reasons. Hopefully, by increasing your strength, balance and posture, we can get you moving unaided again. If not, you'll still have got into the habit of doing a little daily exercise, which will benefit your overall health and wellbeing.

Each week, we will focus on a different area of the body. We will use short, gentle exercises to strengthen your body and work on your balance and coordination. I'll describe exercises that

I would like you to do daily. These daily exercises will work on strengthening your weaknesses and ironing out the imbalances in your body that may be causing your reduced mobility.

My whole ethos is that a little exercise done daily is far better than one big session a week.

So, let's begin our journey and get you moving again, because who says age should slow you down?

Before you start

You have a different set of exercises to do each week. **Do each exercise for that week once a day**.

Activating your core should be the beginning of any movement or action you make. It will protect your back and control your posture, balance and breathing.

So, what is your core?

Think of the core as the mediator of your body. Without it, your muscles will work on their own but will do what they want and fight against themselves. When you activate your core, your muscles work together, and your body begins to fall into alignment, making your movements easier.

Simply put, your core is all the muscles that are involved in stabilising your body. Our bodies are lazy and will always try to find the easiest way to carry out a movement. Quite often, we slouch and stoop and put all of our movement through our backs, which causes pain and problems all over the body.

By using and strengthening your core, you will keep unnecessary pressure out of your spine and keep your body in the correct anatomical position, creating harmony throughout your muscles and, therefore, your movements.

The main aim of this book is to help reduce your risk of falling. A strong and activated core will go a long way in helping to achieve this.

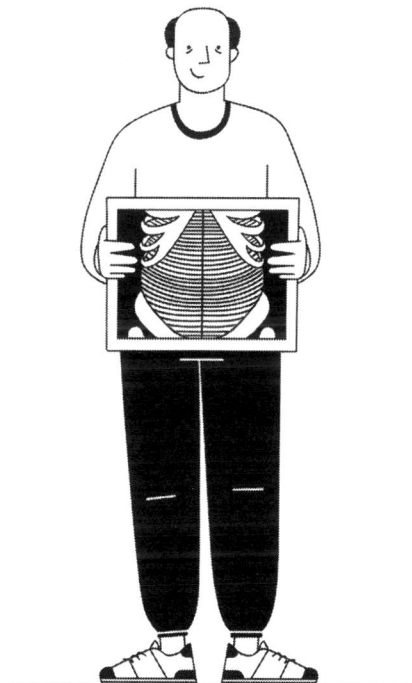

Core 1

➲ Activate your core

Let's begin. The first exercise I want you to do is to discover your core.

► Lie on your back on the bed with your head supported on a pillow. Place your arms down by your sides and your legs out straight.
► Now, place a hand under the arch of your back with the palm facing down onto the bed.
► One leg at a time, bring both legs to a 45-degree angle at the knee with your feet staying flat on the bed. You will now be lying on your back with your knees bent. As you bring your knees up, you should feel the arch in your lower back decreasing and your spine putting more pressure on your hand.

Lying on your back with your knees bent puts your spine into a neutral position. When you lie on your back with your legs out straight, the weight of your legs lifts and arches your back, putting unnecessary pressure into the spine. By lying with bent knees, you are hitting the reset button and taking the pressure out of your lower back.

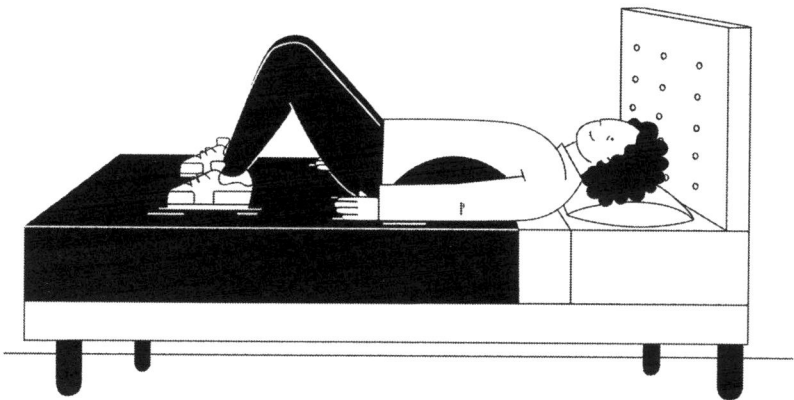

This is a great tip for those days when your back is causing you pain and you are struggling for relief. Just lie on the bed with bent knees for 10 minutes and hit the reset button. As you lie, the muscles around your spine will relax and should help to ease the muscle spasm that causes the back pain.

Now let's find your core. There are many core muscles so, to simplify things, we are going to start with just one, the transversus abdominis (TVA).

➲ Find your TVA

- Lying on your back with your knees bent, feet flat on the bed, place both your index fingers on your navel.
- Move them an inch down towards your legs and then run them across to your hips, stopping before you reach the pelvis or when you can feel bone.
- Take in a breath and, as you exhale, pull your belly button in and draw it up towards your chest. Press your fingertips down so you can feel the muscle activating. Hold for 10 seconds.
- Repeat no more than five times.

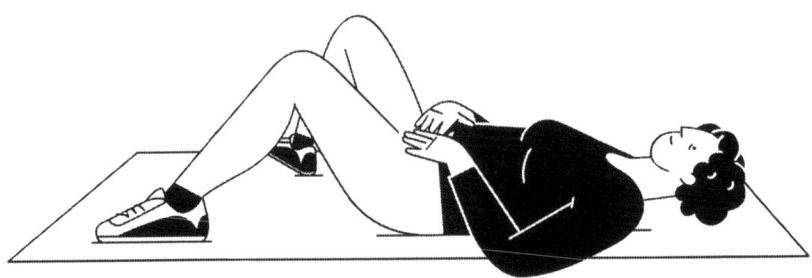

It might take a few attempts to feel this as the muscle is deep and there may not be an obvious contraction. You are trying to feel a deep muscle tightening as you push down with your fingertips. When you can feel it, hold the contraction for a few seconds, whilst remembering to breathe.

I want you to do this exercise every day this week. It is easy to overdo this exercise, which can lead to a strain, so do not do it more than once a day, for a maximum of five holds, and hold for no more than 10 seconds each time. By the end of the week, we are aiming for you to be able to recognise your TVA, which I'll call your core, and know exactly how to activate it.

Core 2

➲ Pelvic floors

Pelvic floors are another core muscle group and they work together with the TVA. As we age, the pelvic floors weaken, like all other muscles. This exercise will help strengthen your core and will also improve bladder control.

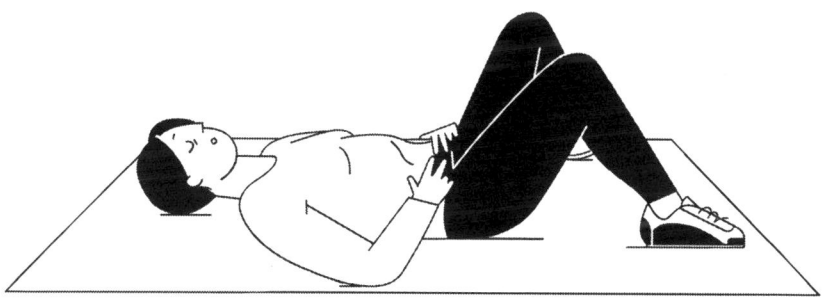

- ▶ Lie on your back with your knees bent, feet flat on the bed.
- ▶ The best way to explain how to do this is to think about tightening your internals. Imagine you are holding in a wee. Try not to hold your breath.

▶ Now isolate your internal muscles without tightening your buttocks and stomach. Squeeze those muscles 10 times in a row.

▶ When you are used to doing it, try holding each squeeze for a few seconds. It is easy to overdo this exercise so don't go for it. Rest for a few seconds between each squeeze!

➲ Single leg heels off

Here we will really put some strength into your core muscles.

▶ Lie on your back, knees bent, feet flat on the bed with your arms by your sides. With a neutral spine engage your core. Try not to strain, but pull in just enough to feel your muscles.

▶ Now, using one leg, keep your heel on the bed and raise your toes.

▶ Making sure you keep your core on, raise your heel slightly off the bed, about the height of a closed fist. When doing this, keep your knee in the same position so the exercise comes from your hip.

▶ Lower your heel and repeat the lift 10 times. Then do the exercise with the other leg.

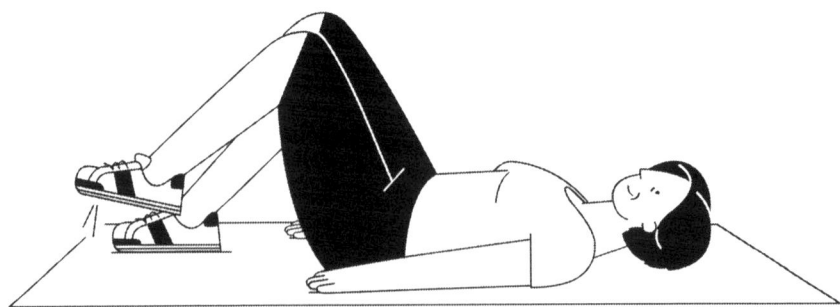

Core 3

➲ Sit with engaged core

With this exercise, the height of the chair is vital. If the chair is too low, your bottom will be below your knees, which tilts your pelvis and puts unwanted pressure into your back.

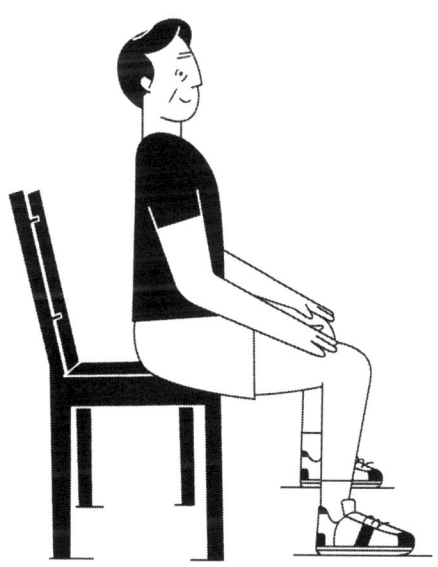

- ▶ Sit on a chair with your feet hip distance apart, knees at a 90-degree angle so your heels are directly under your knees. Try to avoid using the back of the chair, and sit up straight with an open chest.
- ▶ Now, as you did in week one, engage your core by activating your TVA. Try to keep your shoulders relaxed and your eyes facing forward. Remember to breathe.

Before you have mastered the art of isolating the individual muscles required, you will probably 'hit and hope'. We all tend to pull in everything in the beginning, but everything will include your diaphragm. This will basically stop you breathing, so just check with yourself every now and then that you are still drawing in a breath.

Try to hold this for 10 seconds the first time, then increase the hold by 10 seconds each day. By the end of the week I would like you to be able to sit there and hold for 1 minute. Don't be tempted to try this exercise more than three times in one session as overdoing it can cause a strain.

When you start getting used to sitting with an engaged core, you can try working on the amount of force you are using to activate it. Instead of pulling in as hard as you can using 100% effort, activate your core and then reduce the effort by 50%. When that feels under control, reduce that effort by a further 50% and hold. You will now be sitting there with the ideal amount of sustainable effort activating your core. It's at this level that you can realistically aim to keep your core on all day without the worry of injury.

Stop being top-heavy

This will increase your balance and reduce your risk of falls.

The average human head weighs around 5kg. If your posture is good, your head will rest nicely on top of your neck with all of its weight evenly distributed throughout your body. Unfortunately, that's not what most of us do. We slouch, stoop and walk with our eyes to the floor, which makes us top-heavy.

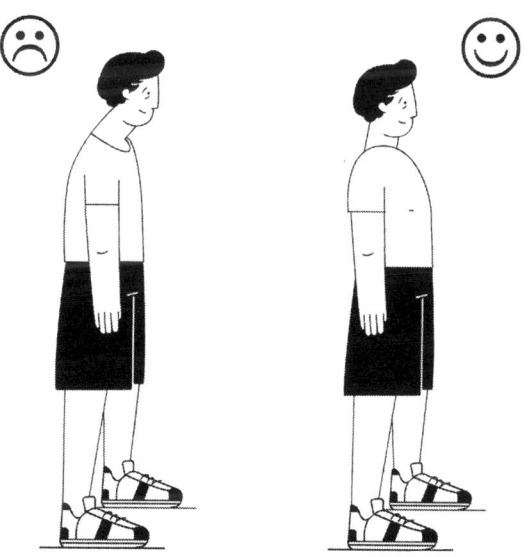

If your eyes are looking down, your head and neck are bent forwards, which puts an increased curve in your upper spine. This pushes your shoulders and chest forward, making your body weight off balance. If you trip, there is only one way you will go, and your 5kg of head will lead the way. If your core is on and your posture is good, you are much less likely to fall, and if you do trip, you will be more likely to hold your balance.

This week we will try to correct this by loosening your shoulders. However, this is not a quick fix. The chances are that your body has been in this position for years and it will take more than one week of shoulder circles to correct the poor posture. You will get there. Just be mindful of the position of your head by looking straight in front of you when you do this exercise.

➲ Shoulder circles

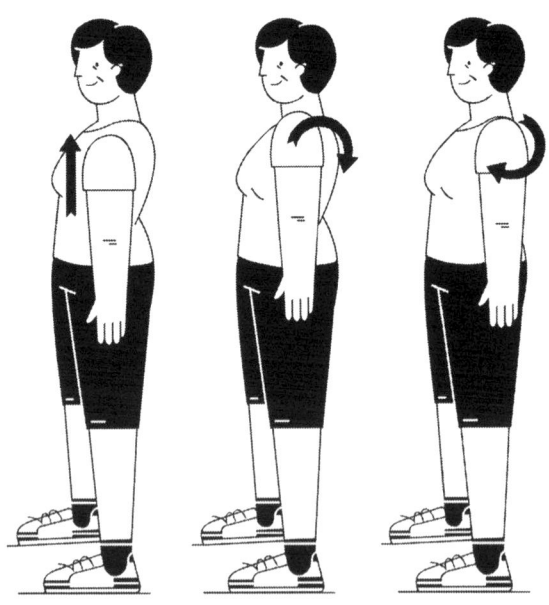

- Stand tall with your core activated, feet hip distance apart. With your arms straight down by your sides, fix your gaze on something directly in front of you.
- Keeping your arms straight to focus the movement in your shoulders, raise your shoulders as high as you can then roll them back behind you in a circular motion. Roll your shoulders back 10 times, trying to increase the movement each time, and don't forget about your core!

You may feel and hear a lot of crunching and cracking going on in your upper back. Don't worry, as this is quite normal. Muscle is a soft tissue but when it's tight and tense the fibres stick together forming solid lumps of tissue. This is what you can hear as you roll: all the muscle fibres around the shoulder blade unsticking and coming apart. So, the more crunching, the merrier!

Open your chest and ribs

➲ Deep breathing

Now we are going to start to open your chest and rib cage, which can hold a lot of compression that you may not be aware of.

► I want you to go back to the exercise in week 3 and sit with an engaged core. As you do it, take big, deep breaths in through your nose and out through your mouth.

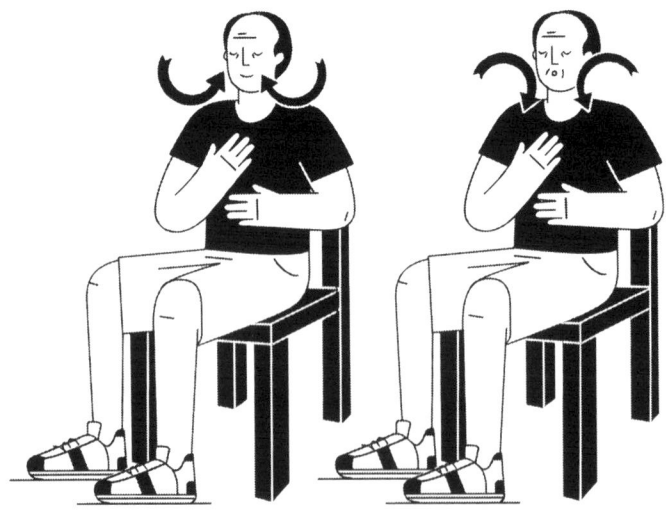

- ▶ Really focus on your lungs filling up with oxygen. Feel your chest expanding and your rib cage opening. Avoid taking in shallow breaths by counting to four as you inhale and again when you exhale.
- ▶ Try to switch off your thoughts and relax your mind. Imagine the air going into your lungs and into your bloodstream, being transported all around your body. Oxygen is life and you are supplying it to every part of yourself.
- ▶ Do this for 1 minute, trying to increase to 2 minutes by the end of the week.

Strengthen your upper back

➲ Shoulder blade squeeze

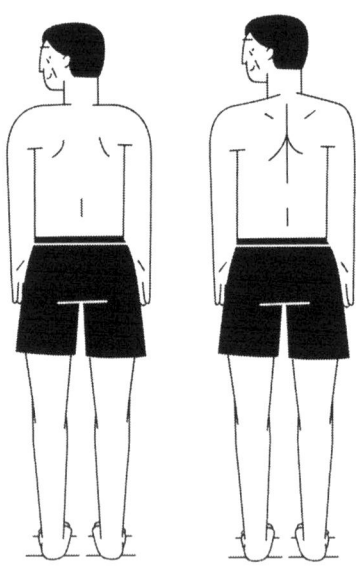

This exercise will strengthen the big muscles in your upper back that will help you to avoid being top-heavy.

▶ Stand or sit with your core engaged and eyes facing forward.

▶ Place your arms by your sides in a relaxed position, shoulders down.

▶ Moving your shoulders as little as possible, try to squeeze your shoulder blades together. Hold for 5 seconds, relax, then try again.

▶ Repeat this cycle 10 times.

Keep your chest open

After activating your core, I believe maintaining an open chest is the next most important action you should think about. When the large muscles of the chest tighten, they pull your shoulders and head forward, making you stoop and become top-heavy and increasing your risk of falling. When I'm treating clients who complain of headaches and neck ache, by far the main reason for this is a tight chest. A tight chest will pull your shoulders forward and, as a consequence, the weight of your arms will hang from your neck instead of your shoulder joints. This overworks the muscles, creating tension and subsequently pain.

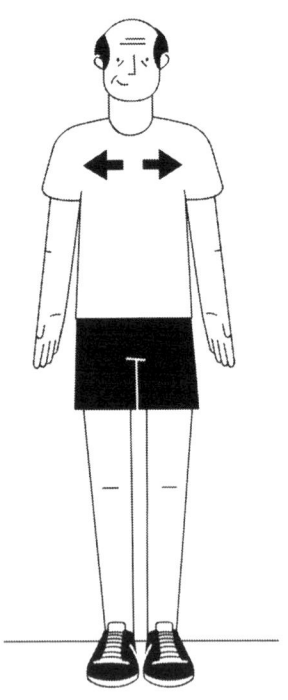

The chest muscles run from your sternum all the way to your upper arm. To open your chest, ease your shoulders back. Be mindful when opening your chest not to arch your lower back, which is easy to do.

To feel your chest opening, you should first feel your rib cage expanding and your shoulders gently travelling back. The best way to try this is to take in a breath and, as you exhale, open your ribs and feel the muscles of the chest lifting. Try not to force your shoulders back. If you do this you can easily pull a muscle you didn't know was tight. When opening your chest, activate you core and get them both working together. I want you to be mindful of this all week. Whatever you are doing, do it with an open chest!

➲ Chest stretch

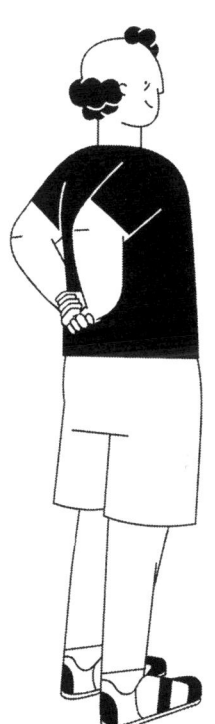

Now let's try to stretch your chest muscles. You can do this standing or sitting.

- ▶ Stand or sit tall with a neutral spine, feet hip distance apart. Open your chest and relax your shoulders. Activate your core.
- ▶ Make fists behind you in the small of your back and gently try to bring your elbows together behind you, and then your shoulder blades.
- ▶ Hold for 20 seconds, taking in big breaths as you do. Breathe in through your nose and out through your mouth. Keep your eyes facing forward, trying not to bend your neck.

You will feel your chest muscles stretching from your sternum towards your shoulders. You may also feel something in your shoulders as they stretch, but look out for pain. If your shoulders are too tight or carrying an injury, the stretch will aggravate it, so be careful.

Balance your quads and hamstrings

Most people have an imbalance in their thigh muscles. The quadriceps are the four muscles in the front of the thigh and the hamstrings are the three muscles in the back. As there are more muscles in the front, you would expect them to be stronger than those at the back. I would be happy if your quads were around 20% stronger than your hamstrings, but in most people it's more like 50%. We tend to work our quads much more than our hamstrings, which creates the imbalance.

If you have this imbalance it can cause lower back pain, which will affect your posture and walking ability. As your quad muscles overtighten, they pull on the front of your pelvis tilting it forward. This weakens the hamstrings and puts pressure into your lower back. If your hamstring muscles are already weak, they will let your pelvis rise even more. You are then left with an imbalance all around your hip muscles, which will create pain and instability.

Over the next two weeks, we will learn how to fix this problem.

➲ Hamstring stretch

Tight hamstring muscles can be a cause of back pain all on their own. As you sit, you naturally shorten these muscles, so the longer you sit, the tighter they become.

▸ First of all, lie on your back, feet flat on the bed with your knees bent. Maintaining a neutral spine, lower your right leg so it is flat on the bed.
▸ Keep your core muscles activated and breathe in. As you exhale, gently raise your right leg off the bed until you feel a stretch. Hold the stretch for 20 to 30 seconds and feel the muscles easing off.
▸ Lower it back down and repeat with the other leg.

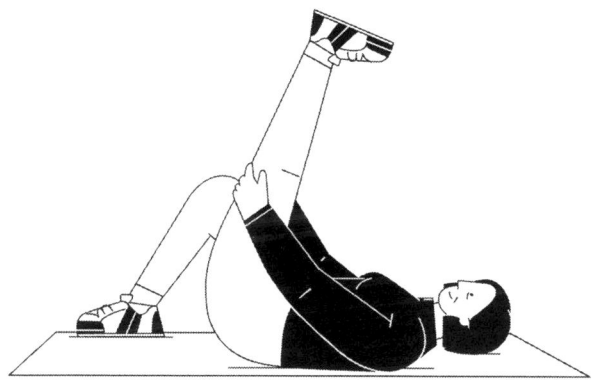

Don't force it, and try to keep the rest of your body relaxed. At this stage it doesn't matter if your leg is straight or bent. Your muscles will tell you how far and how much you can stretch. Listen to them. If you can feel a massive pull in the back of your leg or it is shaking then that is enough. If there is hardly any sensation then try placing your hands behind your knee and gently guide your leg towards you by pulling with your hands, increasing the stretch.

⮕ Quad stretch

If you've had a knee replacement then do not do this stretch.
An alternative is an exercise commonly given during rehabilitation: sitting in a chair, draw your foot back towards your body so your knee gets to at least a 90-degree angle. Hold it there for 20 seconds then let go of the stretch, relaxing your thigh.

You will need a tea towel for this exercise.

▸ Take the tea towel and place it around your right ankle. Lie on your front. Keep your head down so you do not strain your neck.
▸ Using your right arm, pull the tea towel towards your bottom, bending your knee. Keep your knees touching and your chest down on the bed.
▸ When you can feel a stretch in the front of your thigh and you can't pull any more, gently push your hips into the bed. This will intensify the stretch and you should feel a strong pull in the quads.
▸ Hold the stretch for 20 seconds then repeat with the other leg. The aim is to get your foot as near to your bottom as possible.

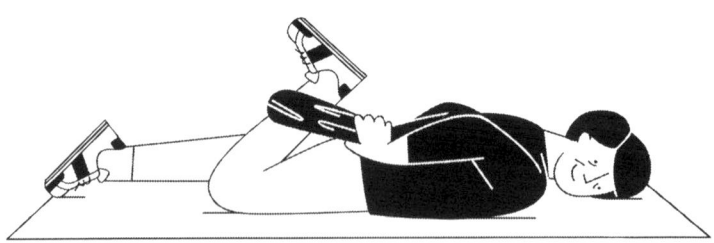

Strengthen your thighs

➲ Bridge

This exercise will strengthen your hamstrings and start to address the imbalance between the front and back of your thigh muscles.

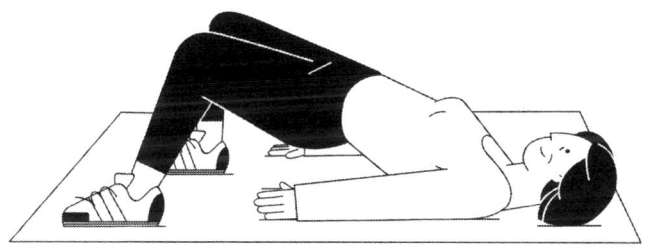

▸ Lie on your back with your knees bent, feet hip distance apart, arms by your sides. Take in a few deep breaths, relaxing your upper body.
▸ Engage your core and, maintaining a neutral spine, take in a breath. As you exhale, use your core and lift your bottom off the bed, placing your body weight onto your shoulder blades. Tighten your buttocks to lock the position.
▸ Hold the bridge position for 20 seconds.

You will feel a pull on the muscles at the back of your thigh. If you feel anything stronger than a pull, like the muscles beginning to cramp, gently lower yourself down and stretch your hamstrings before trying again.

Rebalance your quads

➲ Straight leg raises

Before you do this exercise, you need to learn about the midline. Imagine drawing a line straight down the centre of your thigh. Start at the top, go down the centre, pass through the centre of your knee and down into your middle toe.

You need to visualise the midline for this exercise to make sure that the four quad muscles are worked evenly. If the midline is off, this will add to your imbalance. If your toes are facing away from your body instead of in line with the midline, you will isolate the inner thigh muscles; and if your toes are facing towards your body, you will work the outside of the thigh.

As you are striving for balance in your thighs, you need to have your toes central and vertical.

▶ Lie on your back with your knees bent, feet flat on the bed. Straighten one leg and place a rolled-up towel under that knee. You do this to make sure you don't overextend your knee, which will pull the muscles behind it.
▶ In order to maintain a neutral spine, the leg you are not using should stay bent at a 45-degree angle, with your foot flat on the bed. This helps prevent you arching your back as you raise your leg.

► Keep your hands by your sides and make sure your neck is comfortable. Using the straight leg, point your toes towards your body to activate the calf and lock your leg into position.

► Make sure your leg is in the correct position using the midline and activate your core. Take in a breath and, as you exhale, raise your leg off the bed a few centimetres and hold it there for 10 seconds, checking that the midline is still correct and remembering to breathe.

► After the 10 seconds, gently lower and do it again with the same leg. Remember not to arch your back, and keep checking your core is on.

► Repeat this 5 to 10 times depending on how much you can cope with, then do exactly the same with the other leg.

Don't overdo it. This exercise is as much about being able to maintain your core as it is lifting your leg in the air.

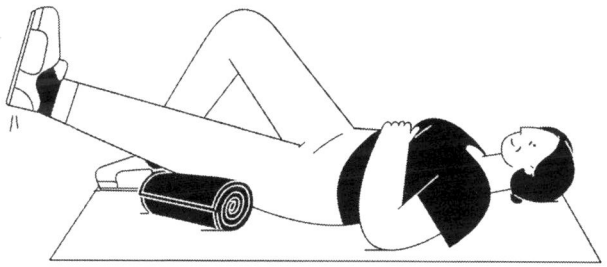

Loosen your ankles and strengthen your calves

➲ Plantarflex/dorsiflex

Plantarflex means point your toes away from you and dorsiflex means point your toes towards you. You can do this exercise either sitting or lying on the bed.

▸ Point your toes away from you (plantarflex), holding for a second, then point your toes towards you (dorsiflex).
▸ Plantarflex and dorsiflex 20 times with each foot.

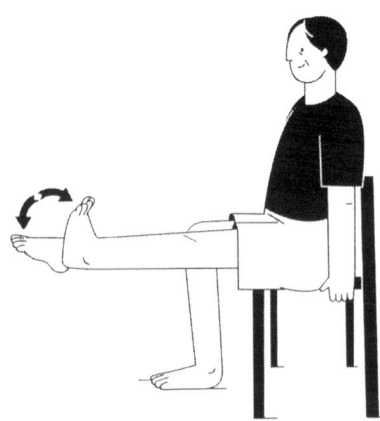

As your toes travel towards you, your calf muscles (in the back of the leg between the ankle and the knee) will tighten. How much your foot moves is completely dependent on the amount of tension present in your calf. The looser the calf, the more movement you will have in your foot.

⮕ Ankle rotations

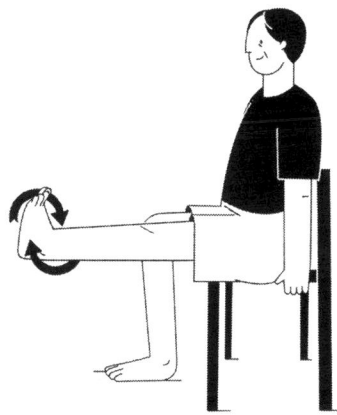

► Seated or lying on the bed, rotate your foot at the ankle 10 times in one direction and then 10 times in the other.

Was that a nice smooth action with no restriction and full range, or was it sore or hesitant? In order to seek out knots and deal with tension, you can look for hesitation. If your muscles are absolutely fine there won't be any. It is imbalance, weakness and tension that cause hesitation by putting stress on the way the muscles move. The muscles end up fighting against what should be a natural action, causing hesitation.

► Try the ankle rotation again in both directions, aiming for a smooth, full movement.

⮞ Calf raises

► Stand with your arms straight out in front of you at shoulder height and your palms lightly touching a wall for support. Your feet should be hip distance apart, and your heels and toes equal distance apart (feet parallel).

► Engage your core and breathe in. As you exhale, push off your heels onto your toes and hold for a second, then come back down.

► Don't rush. Ease up and down, holding for a second at the top. Repeat 10 times.

Try to keep the pressure in the balls of your feet. You don't want to push up too high and end up with too much pressure on your toes. Aim to keep your feet square, heels and toes the same distance apart.

Quite often, because of problems elsewhere, the heels start moving inwards, towards themselves. That will not work the muscle fibres in the calf evenly, resulting in an imbalance.

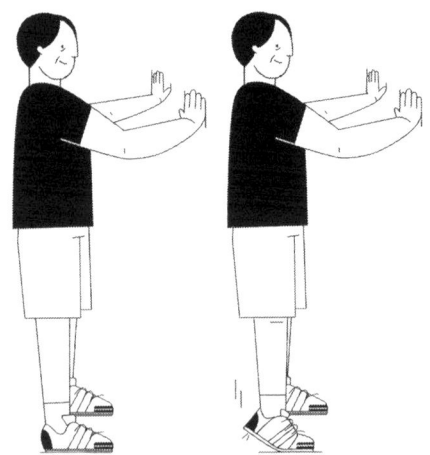

Loosen your hips and bum

It is important to keep your hips and bottom loose to maintain mobility. If your muscles are loose, they will allow greater movement without straining and your walking will flow. These muscles are some of the largest in the body and are the source of 90% of back pain in the clients I treat.

➲ Chair trunk twists

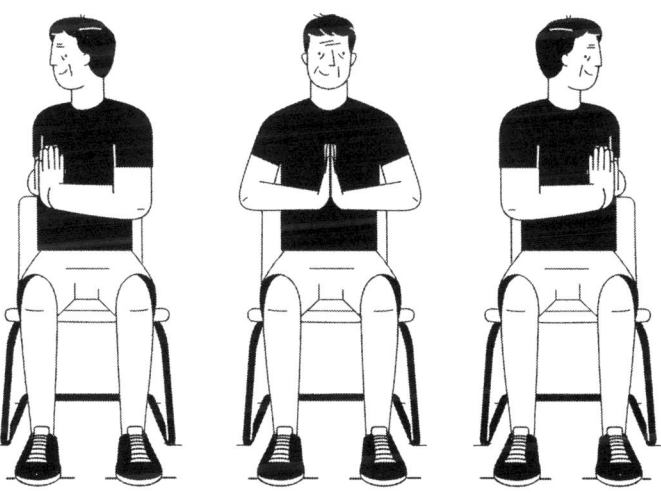

▸ Sit with your feet hip distance apart and activate your core. Raise your arms so they are shoulder height, then bend your elbows 90 degrees with fingertips touching. Your upper arms should now be parallel to the floor.

▸ Anchor your feet to the floor and try not to move your legs. Holding this position, and keeping your neck still, twist from your waist as far as you can with your head, arms and torso moving together as one.

▸ Come back to the centre and then twist over to the other side. Keep the movement slow and controlled, holding the twist for a few seconds before you return to the centre.

▸ Repeat this five times on each side.

➲ Legs out to the side

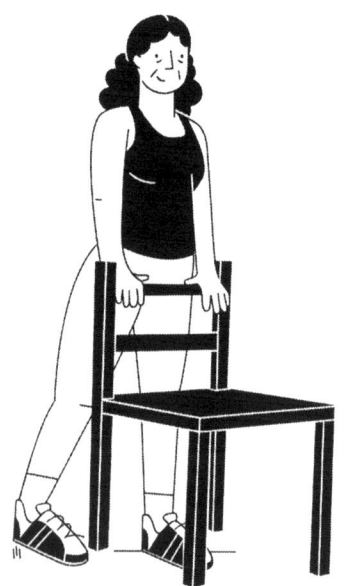

▸ Standing tall with something sturdy to hold on to, activate your core. Open your chest and keep your shoulders relaxed, eyes forward.

▸ Keeping your leg as straight as possible without tilting your body, raise one leg out to the side, just enough to lift it off the floor. You should feel the muscles working around the hip of your active leg.

▸ Keep the leg that stays on the floor still. Try to feel the foot of that leg pressing into the floor, with your body weight going evenly down through the leg into your heel and the ball of your foot.

▸ Repeat five times with each leg.

➲ Clam

▶ Lie on your side with a pillow or your arms supporting your head. Straighten your legs, with your hips and shoulders in a straight line.

▶ Bend your knees so that your lower legs are at a 90-degree angle to your body. Make sure your knees do not travel forwards, keeping them in line with your chest.

▶ Making sure you have a neutral spine and your core is activated, tilt your hips slightly forward. If you don't do this, as you begin the exercise, your back will try to take over and you will lose alignment.

▶ Keep your feet together and lift your top knee only, opening your legs. Then slowly lower the knee back to the start position. Only go as far as you can whilst keeping your core on and maintaining alignment.

▶ Do this exercise 10 times on each side.

The golden rule of the clam is that your hips can never be too far forward. This keeps the exercise out of your back and into the gluteus medius. If the movement is big, you are doing it wrong. You should feel this in the muscle just behind your hip in the buttock of your top leg.

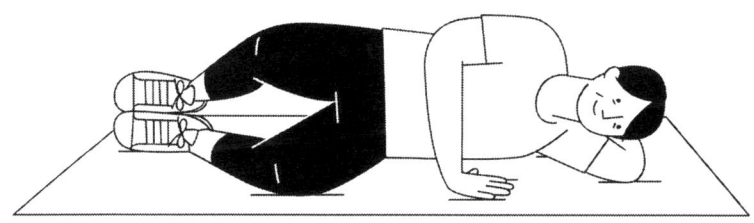

Work on your balance

➲ Kitchen side steps

The purpose of this exercise is to strengthen your hips and work on your balance.

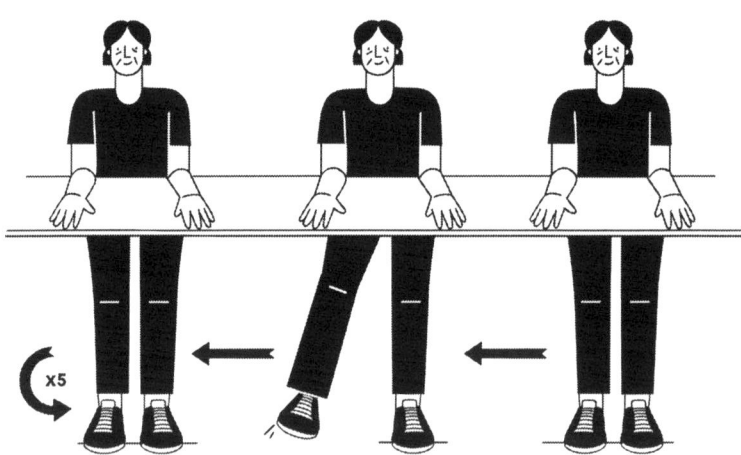

▶ Gently rest both hands on a solid kitchen surface, activate your core and open your chest. Make sure your feet are hip distance apart. This is the closest they should be during this exercise.

▶ Take five steps to the side keeping your hips forward and your knees soft, moving your hands along the surface as you go. As you step, make sure your feet do not come together. Keep them hip distance apart for stability.

▶ When you have finished stepping one way, repeat the other way, again taking five sideways steps. Keep going until you have done this five times each side.

➲ One foot forward, heel off

▶ Stand tall with your feet hip distance apart and soften your knees. Activate your core and open your chest. You may want to use the kitchen surface again for support depending on your balance abilities.

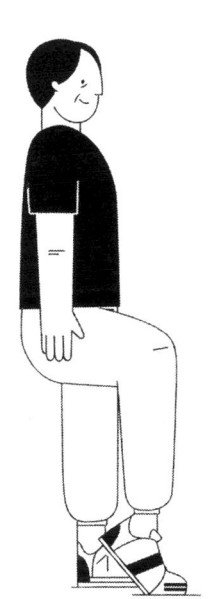

▶ With your feet staying hip distance apart, take a little step forward with one foot. Make sure the heel of the foot you have stepped with doesn't travel past the toes of your stationary foot.

▶ Keeping your chest open and spine neutral, raise the heel of the forward foot off the floor, keeping your toes grounded.

▶ Try to feel the calf and thigh of that leg doing the work. In the stationary leg, try to feel your body weight is evenly distributed straight down the centre of the leg into the whole of your foot.

▶ Hold that position for at least 10 seconds whilst breathing and staying relaxed.

▶ Repeat on the other side.

Improve your posture

➲ One foot forward, knee to waist

The first time you do this exercise, place one hand on the kitchen surface for support. The second time, just use your fingertips for light support. When you feel confident with the exercise, try doing it without holding on, using your core to stabilise your body. This balance exercise goes a long way to helping you walk unaided.

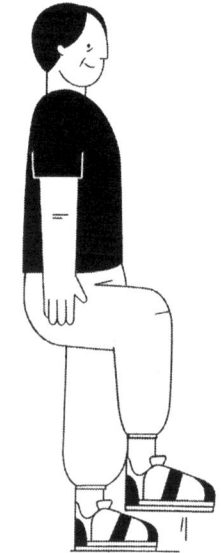

- ▶ As before, with the heel off exercise, stand tall with an open chest, feet hip distance apart.
- ▶ Keeping your feet at that distance apart, take a little step forward with one foot. Make sure the heel of the foot you have stepped with doesn't travel past the toes of your stationary foot.
- ▶ Keeping your chest open and spine neutral, raise the heel of the forward foot off the floor, keeping your toes grounded.

▸ Try to feel the calf and thigh of that leg doing the work. In the stationary leg, try to feel your body weight is evenly distributed straight down the centre of the leg into the whole of your foot.

▸ Hold that position for a few seconds then, without tilting into your hip, raise your leg up so your knee is waist high at a 90-degree angle. Try to hold it there, perfectly still, for 10 seconds.

▸ Lower back to the start then repeat with the other leg.

➲ Dip with the knees

This exercise will strengthen your thighs and help improve your posture.

▸ Stand facing the kitchen surface with your hands palm down on top to support your body weight. You will be bending your knees so you want to make sure there is a sufficient distance between you and the kitchen unit to do this.

▸ Place your feet hip distance apart, activate your core and open your chest.

▸ Gently lower your body by bending your knees. Don't go down too far, just enough to feel your thigh muscles working.

▸ Really concentrate on keeping your back straight by looking directly ahead and maintaining a neutral spine.

▸ Repeat this 10 times.

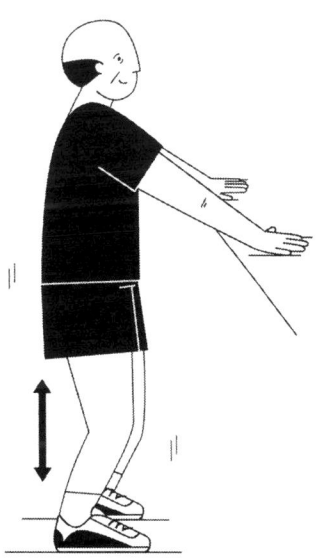

Increase your balance

➲ Box step

This is a great exercise to increase your balance and coordination.

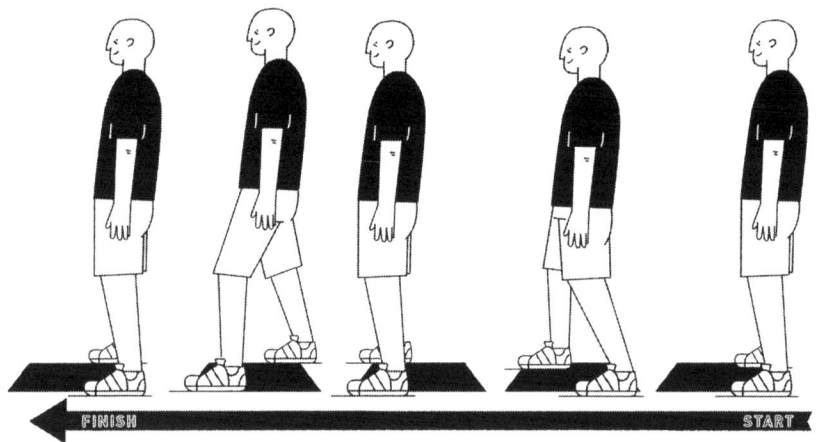

- ► Stand tall, with your feet hip distance apart. Use some support the first time you do this until your confidence has grown and you feel secure without holding on.
- ► Starting with your right foot, take a step forward, making sure to hit the floor with your heel first, followed by your toes.

▸ Then bring your left foot forward level with the right, keeping them hip distance apart.

▸ Next, step your right foot back to the start position, landing on your toes first and then the heel. Keeping your feet hip distance apart, step your left leg back to its start position.

▸ This is a box step: think right, left, right left and forward, forward, back, back.

▸ Repeat this sequence 10 times then do it again but starting with your left foot.

Use your new strength

Now we are going to practise putting everything together. This will get your body working in harmony, as a complete unit. You are aiming for ease of movement that's unrestricted and without hesitation. Achieving this will give you better freedom of movement, making you sturdier on your feet.

➲ Stand with your core on

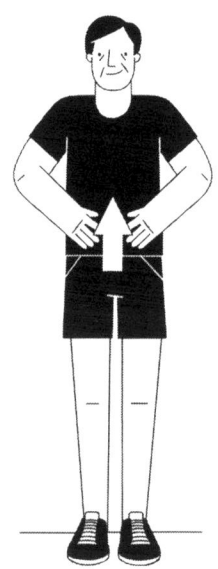

▸ Stand with your feet hip distance apart with soft knees. Activate your core and be mindful of a neutral spine.
▸ Place your arms by your sides and open your chest. Keep looking straight ahead, and stand upright so you can feel your ribs are open and not compressed.
▸ Now, as you did in week one, engage your core by activating your TVA. Remember, you don't want to strain it, just activate it like in week 3.
▸ If you need more practice, pull in strongly and then reduce the effort by 50%. When that feels under control, reduce that effort by a further 50% and hold.

- Stand in this position for 30 seconds, taking slow, big breaths in through your nose and out through your mouth.
- During this week's exercise sessions, try to increase the hold by 30 seconds at a time until you can stand with your core on for 2 minutes without interruption.

➲ Arm swings

- As before, stand with your feet hip distance apart with soft knees. Activate your core and be mindful of a neutral spine.
- Place your arms by your sides and open your chest. Keep looking straight ahead, and stand upright so you can feel your ribs are open and not compressed.
- Keeping your arms straight and fingers together, not splayed, swing your arms, alternating one arm back and one forward as you do. When your arm goes forward, bring it up level with your chest. When it goes back, aim for waist height.
- Do this continuously for 30 seconds.

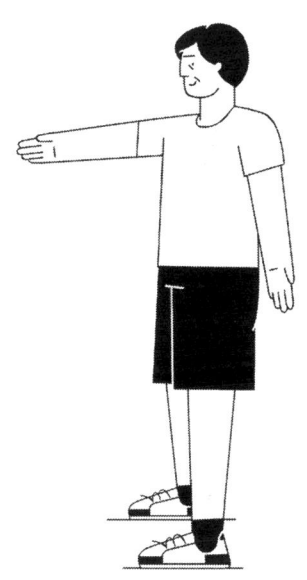

You will notice as you swing your arms that your hips rock from side to side. This is because your arm movement is prompting hip swing, which is what will make your walking flow and help you be much more energy efficient.

➲ Chair sit-ups

First of all, you need to find the correct chair. The height of the chair is just as important as the exercise itself. When seated, your bottom should be level with or slightly higher than your knees. Place the chair next to a wall so that it can't slip backwards during this exercise.

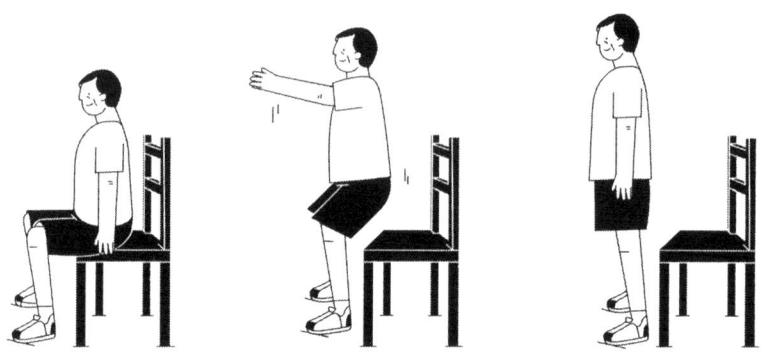

- ▶ Start by sitting on the chair, a few centimetres away from the back – just enough so that your back is not touching the chair.
- ▶ Activate your core and make sure your spine is neutral. Place your arms down by your sides. Keep your eyes facing forward, fixed on something in front of you.
- ▶ With your feet hip distance apart and toes very slightly facing out, stand up from the chair slowly and feel your thighs and bottom muscles working. You should also feel your stomach muscles tighten. You should not feel anything in your back.
- ▶ As you stand, try not to lock your knees, keeping them soft. Stand tall for a moment, feeling your body weight is evenly distributed down each thigh and into your feet.

▸ Take in a breath and, as you exhale, lower yourself back into the chair by pushing your bottom back whilst keeping your spine neutral and your core activated.

▸ Repeat this exercise five times. Don't rush, and take big breaths throughout.

Make sure your eyes stay looking forward and you don't look down. Also, be aware of what your knees are doing. It's absolutely normal for your body to try to cheat. This usually happens with your knees moving towards each other. It's a normal habit in which your mind is telling your body that you are better off doing so. Be aware of this and keep your knees equal distance apart throughout the entire exercise.

Make sure that your knees don't travel forward past your toes. By keeping them just over your ankles and pushing your bottom back, you will really engage your quads and gluteus muscles, keeping unwanted pressure out of your knees and lower back.

Reach further

➲ Squat and reach

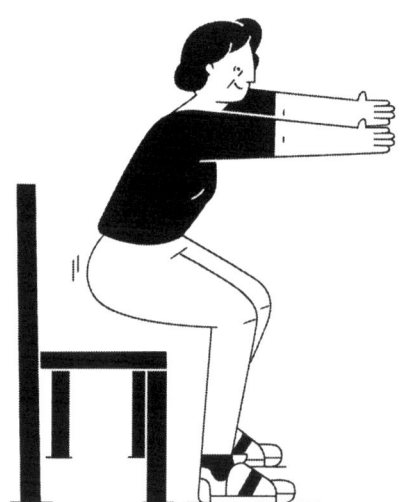

▶ Stand in front of your chair, a few centimetres away from it –
just enough so that the backs of your legs are not touching the
chair. Activate your core and make sure your spine is neutral.

▶ Bend your elbows and place your hands in front of your chest,
elbows behind your hands. Keep your eyes facing forward,
fixed on something in front of you.

- With your feet hip distance apart, toes very slightly facing out, imagine you are sitting down on the chair and push your bottom as far back as you can.
- At the same time, push your hands forward until your arms are straight.
- As your bottom goes back, your knees will bend. Lower your bottom so that it touches the chair but don't sit down or put your body weight onto the chair. Keep your body weight in your thighs, buttocks and core.
- Pause for a second in the squat, then gently stand back up, bringing your hands back to your chest and bending your elbows.
- Repeat this five times.

Even better balance

➲ March on the spot

▸ Stand tall, feet hip distance apart, open your chest and relax your shoulders.
▸ Activate your core and, with a neutral spine, start marching on the spot. Keep your eyes up as looking down will make you top-heavy and a lot more likely to fall.
▸ Bring your knees up no higher than hip height because any further will arch your back.
▸ Keep your elbows at 90 degrees and swing your arms from the shoulders.
▸ Try not to travel as you are marching. You want to keep to the same position on the floor throughout.

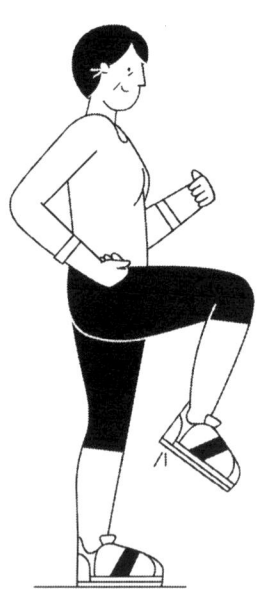

▸ Do this for 30 seconds, taking in big, deep breaths. Breathe in through your nose and out through your mouth. Feel your ribs and chest expanding as you do. Get the oxygen into your body.

➲ Big knee raises

- As before, stand tall with a neutral spine. If you need to, use something sturdy for support.
- With your feet hip distance apart, working one leg at a time, raise your knee slowly to waist height, to the count of three.
- Keeping the angle of your knee at 90 degrees, hold for a few seconds and then gently lower back down whilst also counting to three.
- Repeat the exercise five times with each leg.

You really want to feel the muscles of your core, thigh and hips when you are doing this exercise. You do not want to feel it in your back. If you do, try working on activating your core and make sure your back is staying in a neutral position throughout the exercise.

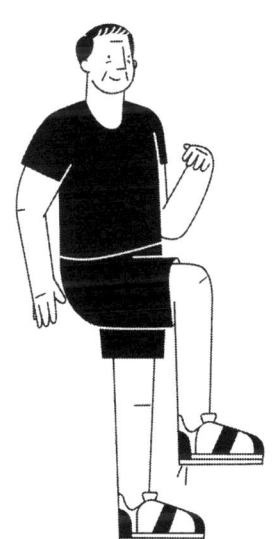

Balance and coordination

➲ Box step with arms

Here we will box step as we did in week 14, but now we will add some arms to increase your balance and coordination.

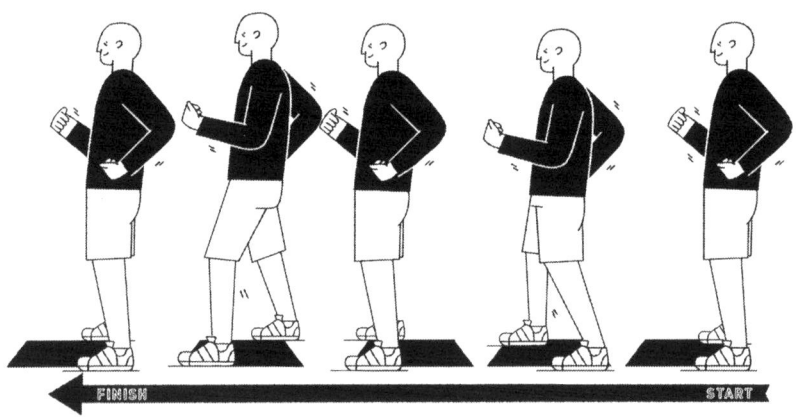

- ► Stand tall, feet hip distance apart. Starting with your right foot, take a step forward, making sure to hit the floor with your heel first, followed by your toes.
- ► Then, bring your left foot forward level with the right, keeping your feet hip distance apart.

- Next, bring your right foot back to the start position, landing on your toes first and then the heel.
- Keeping your feet hip distance apart, step your left leg back to its start position.
- When you have got the rhythm, try adding arm swings into the exercise as you step forward and back. Keep your elbows at a 90-degree angle so your arms do not straighten, and swing your arms from the shoulder.
- Repeat this sequence 10 times then do the same again but starting with your left foot.

➲ Half stars

When you do this exercise, I want you to remember that the closest your feet should be together is hip distance apart. If your feet touch together then you lose your stability.

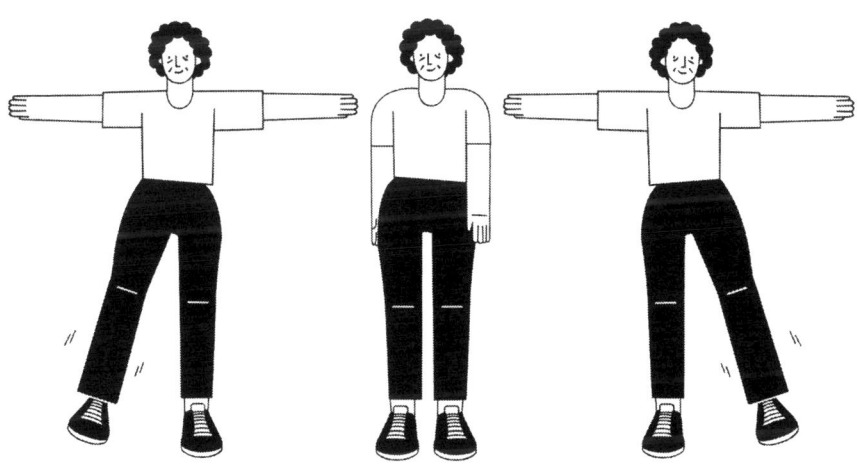

▸ So, with that in mind, stand tall, feet hip distance apart with your core activated and your hands by your sides.

▸ Take a step out to the side with your right leg, tap the toes of your right foot, then bring your foot back to the start.

▸ As you step out, raise both arms out to the side, away from your body to shoulder height, keeping them as straight as you can. When your foot returns to the start, lower your arms.

▸ Do this with the other leg, raising your arms as you step out to the side, lowering your arms as you return your leg to the starting position.

▸ Repeat the sequence, alternating legs 10 times on each side.

Get ready to walk

➲ Heel to toe

Walking heel to toe makes sure your muscles are used effectively and efficiently, putting less tension in them and using less energy. However, when you try it for the first time it may feel wooden and robotic. It is better to practise this one in a corridor with your arms out to the side for balance, using the walls for assistance, or with your stick on hand for safety until it feels more natural.

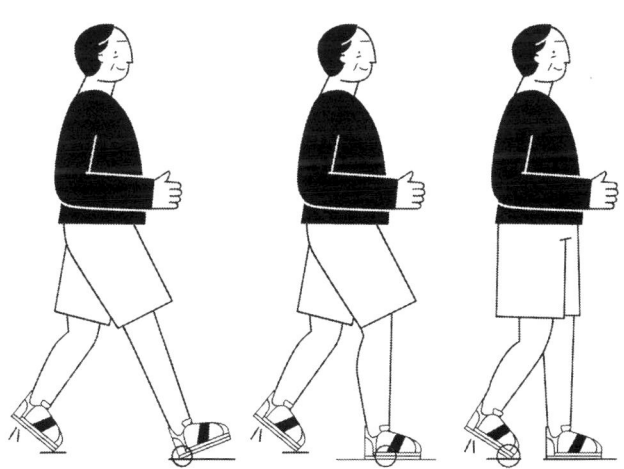

▶ When you are ready, walk heel to toe. Concentrating on each foot in turn, make sure that you strike the ground with your heel first.

▶ Feel the pressure roll towards the balls of your feet then push off with your toes.

▶ Practise this, walking around your home until it feels completely natural.

It might feel like you are walking on the moon but this exercise gets you to roll your body weight through all of your foot. This action will give you more stability and take unnecessary pressure out of your hips, calves, ankles and lower back, enabling you to walk further with greater rhythm.

Power up your walk

➲ Interval walking

Before you start trying to walk outside, I think it is sensible to do the first few trial runs with someone to help you or give an arm should you need it whilst continuing to use your stick or walker. If having your stick makes you feel confident, try carrying it as you walk so that it's there just in case. If you use a walker, take your stick with you and see how your walking feels. If you feel confident to try without the walker, with someone to help support you, try using the stick to walk. Remember, your safety is the primary concern so you must work within your own ability. Don't rush, just progress naturally.

▸ First of all, I want you to walk for 5 minutes as a warm-up. Walk at a gentle pace, heel to toe with your core activated.
▸ Try to keep your head up and chest open, and be mindful that your arms are moving, not stuck down by your sides.

Next you are going to implement interval training. This is a really simple way of increasing your fitness and can be done at any level or ability. During the interval training you will alternate between periods of high intensity and low intensity.

During the high-intensity phase, you will work out in your aerobic zone, walking a little faster than normal, working your heart and lungs. In the period of low intensity, you will recover, walking at a slow, controlled pace. As your fitness improves, you can increase the high-intensity phase and reduce the recovery phase, but for now let's keep it simple.

There are three ways to increase the intensity during a walk.

► Walk up steps
► Walk up an incline
► Walk faster

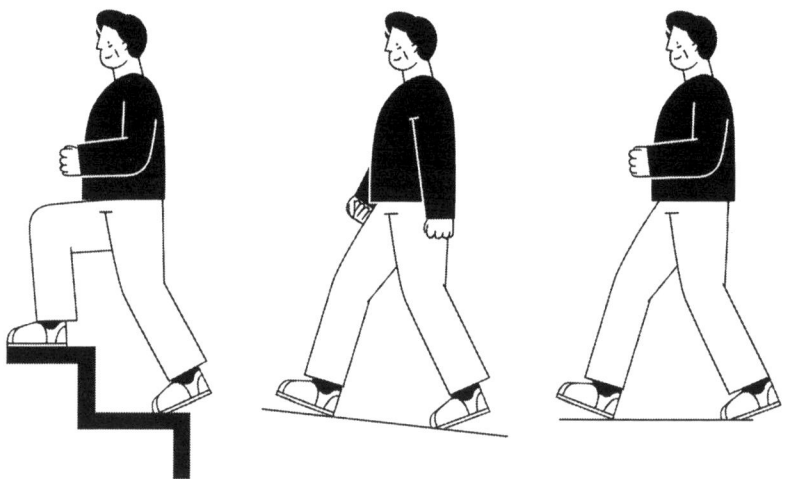

► After the 5-minute warm up, depending on your ability, body issues or confidence, increase the intensity by walking faster or walking up an incline or some steps. Continue doing this for 30 seconds.
► After you have completed the 30 seconds, slow the pace and do recovery walking at low intensity. If you are using steps

or an incline, walk slowly back down. The recovery phase can take as long as you like and will depend on your fitness level. The key is that it's a recovery and that your heart rate goes back down.

▸ When you feel that your heart rate has lowered and you're ready to go again, walk for another 30 seconds at higher intensity.

▸ Repeat this cycle three times: 30 seconds on, then recover.

➲ Power walk

Now you are ready to try a power walk. What I mean by this is that you will walk briskly, in full flight, at pace. The first time you do this it might be a good idea to have someone accompany you until your technique and confidence increase. In the UK, falls are the most common cause of injury-related deaths in people over the age of 75. This statistic really gets to me. With this in mind, make sure that where you are practising is safe to do so, without any trip hazards.

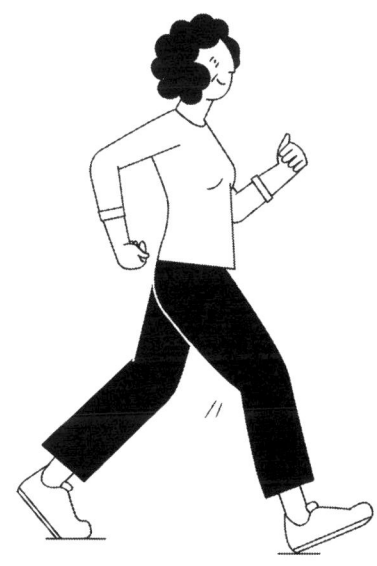

The things to remember when power walking are:

▸ Walk heel to toe, keeping your feet hip distance apart.
▸ Pick up your feet, so you feel that your thighs and hips are working.
▸ Activate your core with a neutral spine.
▸ Keep your chest open and your head up.
▸ Swing your arms.
▸ Take big, deep breaths in through your nose and out through your mouth.

Take command

Well done for reaching the end of this 20-week fitness programme. I know it's a lot to remember, but it will make all the difference to how you walk. After a few attempts it will feel natural. Remember, your body has spent a lifetime developing bad habits. Now it's time to take command and take back control.

Stay safe, stay well and stay MolyFit.

John

www.molyfit.co.uk

Also by the author

A Better You in Later Life

An exercise guide book designed specifically for the over 50s. If you want to stay as active as you can be then exercise is the key. *A Better You in Later Life* is a step-by-step guide to help you recover your strength, balance and mobility. You'll start by learning about posture – the most common problem and usually the cause of most aches and pains. You'll learn how to strengthen your core and maintain a neutral spine. You'll discover how to listen to your body. It's easy to ignore what your body is telling you, and tolerate ongoing pain and discomfort. In *A Better You in Later Life*, you'll learn to re-engage and get moving again using gentle exercise. It may seem strange but you'll re-learn how to walk – putting your body back into the position it should be in, using your muscles in the correct way. You'll also learn how to strengthen and stretch your muscles – dealing with muscular issues you were probably unaware of. Learn how to fix the problem by finding the source and become a better you.

ISBN 978-1-9161271-0-4 (print)

ISBN 978-1-9161271-1-1 (ebook)

https://www.amazon.co.uk/Better-You-Later-Life/dp/191612710X

An Even Better You in Later Life

An 8-week course that gives older adults an easy-to-follow way to partake in daily exercise to improve fitness, health and wellbeing, and to help prevent the common diseases we face in later life.

ISBN 978-1-9161271-2-8 (print)

ISBN 978-1-9161271-3-5 (ebook)

https://www.amazon.co.uk/dp/1916127126

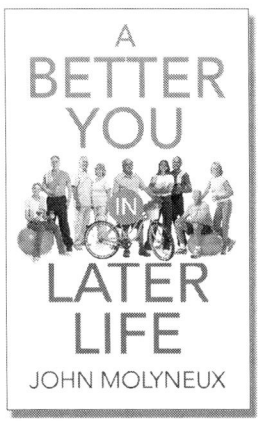
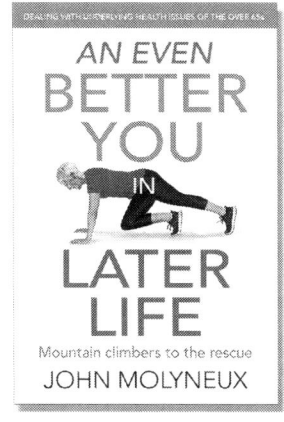

Printed in Great Britain
by Amazon